The Invitation

DAILY LOVE FOR YOUR INTIMATE SELF

Mason & Davis for Rosebud Woman™

ORIGINAL ILLUSTRATIONS BY OUVRA

www.rosebudwoman.com

Special discounts are available on quantity purchases by corporations, associations, and others. For details, contact the publisher at the address above.

Printed in the United States of America

Publisher's Cataloging-in-Publication data

Authors and Contributors:
Mason, Christine Marie. Davis, Carolyn E.. Greenwald, Jeff.

Illustrator: Maria Rozalia Finna (Ouvra)

The Invitation: Daily Love for Your Intimate Self

ISBN-13: 978-0-9977277-6-0

1. Health —Women's Health —Sexuality 2. Self Help—Somatic Healing.

FIRST EDITION

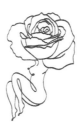

Forgive your mother. Thank her for giving you life
and take it from here. Hell, forgive everyone.

Table of Contents

Table of Illustrations

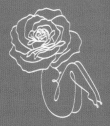

Deep in their roots, all flowers keep the light.
THEODORE ROETHKE

Part 1: An Invitation to Reverence and Awakening

More joy, less suffering.

We created Rosebud Woman because we are in love with everything feminine. We are for more wonder, joy, and delight in every woman's body: especially in the sensitive, delicious, life-and-pleasure-giving design of the area colloquially known as "the pussy." This includes the vulva and vagina, and the surrounding, interconnected structures of the pelvis and pelvic basin.

Yet we know that, for many women, there is pain and discomfort in this area: emotional, mental, somatic, and physical. We know that concerns around lubrication, arousal, irritation, and other elements of the sexual experience exist among women of all ages and in all stages of life. We also realize that sensual pleasure isn't there at the level it could be for everyone—and that these challenges aren't discussed openly. Most women don't even talk with their friends about these issues: they ask the Internet, and sometimes (in less than 10% of cases) a doctor. Why is this so?

Ignoring women's biology reflects a long cultural legacy of downplaying females. There is bias in culture and education, bias in medical research, and bias in the long shadow of religious and political suppression of the feminine. Even the so-called "witch hunts"—which sought out and punished women, especially independent women with knowledge and connection to the plants and wisdom of the earth and its cycles—arose from a fear of the feminine. There's even bias in the language available around what we call a woman's sexual organs. When we were naming the Rosebud Woman balms and potions, we were stunned to see how many words, or euphemisms, had a negative cast, and how they mirrored general insults of the feminine: objectification, judgment, shame, aversion, etc.

Part of this may stem from a more understandable fear of the unknown and the miraculous. It's a miracle even now: You put in semen, and a baby comes out. What dark mystery is this? This reproductive power is something many power structures have sought to regulate and control across many cultures.

And this, in turn, has led to an absence of knowledge, and a lack of self-care. Secrecy leads to suffering: a suffering that doesn't have to be there. We don't take care of the parts that society shuns or shames.

But all of this is changing. We look at our bodies, including the usually ignored parts, and we love and care for them. We learn more about our parts and how they interact. We touch them, we relax them, we strengthen them, we nourish and nurture them. We care for our whole selves, and for our entire personal biome, leaving nothing out.

We also know that nothing exists in isolation.

Our intimate parts rest in the pelvic bowl, which rests in the body, which is infused with blood and all the good and bad materials circulating therein. Our bodies live harnessed to our thoughts, inextricably tied to the earth and the cosmos. So when we look at having a better relationship, more happiness and health in our sex, we have to consider the larger container. It's not just about our genitalia, it's about loving the whole self more.

Changes in the direction of self love may lead to a happier you—and they may also lead to better expression and experiences in the sexual theater. But this is not our primary interest. Our hope is that they will spark a deeper awakening to all the ways you might be in wonder at the miracle of your own body, and cherish yourself more.

Love,

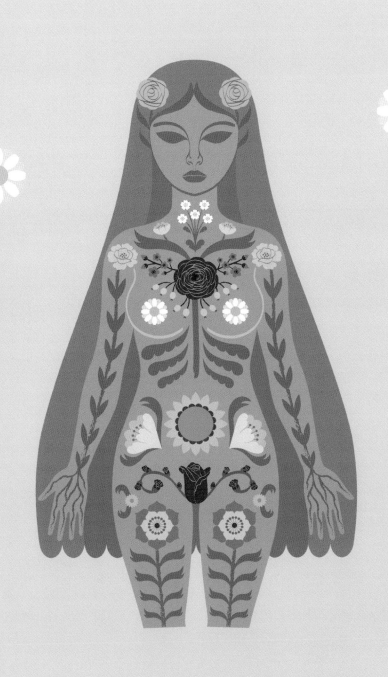

Part 2: Know Your Body Parts

As we talked about in part one, the body is interconnected. Joy, pleasure, and ease in the pelvic and vaginal areas can't be separated from other surrounding systems, or from the body as a whole.

For example, blood flow and nerve transmission in these areas can be impeded by sitting (or by other recurring movement patterns), and by chronic muscle tightening and protections. These will impact the aliveness and sensitivity in the pelvis, and the organs it contains.

We'll be reviewing some self-massage techniques to bring blood flow and relief to the pelvic bowl in Part 4.

To prepare for that, we want to present an overview of the pelvic bowl, and a detailed reveal on the anatomy of the area surrounding the vagina. For some people, this will be a refresher and for some it will be new information. Our images are simple line drawings, and aren't meant to represent an ideal. Like faces, hands or fingerprints, every vagina looks different. We encourage you to take a mirror and look at your own parts, if you haven't already, and get to know your body in its entirety. How do these illustrations compare with your personal anatomy? As we're naming these parts, see if you can locate them on your body.

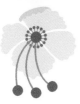

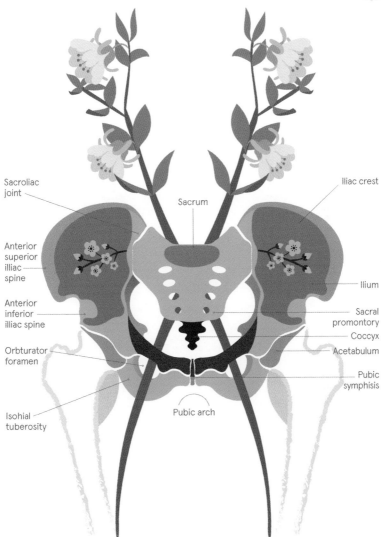

Sacroliac
joint

Sacrum

Iliac crest

Anterior
superior
illiac
spine

Ilium

Anterior
inferior
illiac spine

Sacral
promontory

Orbturator
foramen

Coccyx

Acetabulum

Pubic
symphisis

Isohial
tuberosity

Pubic arch

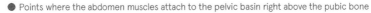

● Points where the abdomen muscles attach to the pelvic basin right above the pubic bone
● Points where the Psoas attaches to the inner thigh
● Pressure points around the top of the pelvis: the iliac ridge and crest.
● Pressure points on the sacrum

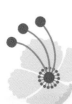
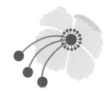

The Bones and Musculature of the Pelvic Bowl

The bones of the pelvis form a basin that supports and contains all of a woman's sexual, reproductive, and elimination organs. This is called the Pelvic Bowl. This area contains a complex net of muscles, ligaments and tendons that connect and help control the torso and the legs, support the back, and influence a person's overall posture.

In the pelvic bowl, we want to draw special attention to four areas that are common causes of discomfort or sensation blockage.

1. The points where the abdomen muscles attach to the pelvic basin, right above the pubic bone. To find them, place your hand on your lower abdomen and do a low sit up. Trace the edges of your abdominal muscles with your fingertips, down to the place they meet the pubic bone. Walk your fingers, using a good amount of pressure, along the pubic bone, pressing down on the top of the bone toward your feet. You will likely feel some tender spots, or pressure points. This is a great place to massage and release tension in the pelvic basin.

2. The points where the Psoas attaches to the inner thigh. The psoas is the only muscle in your body that connects your lower and upper body. It attaches to the middle back, comes down through the pelvis, and attaches to the inner thigh. If it's tight or shortened, it will cause your pelvis to tilt, and impinge blood flow. To work on this spot, bring one knee to your chest, holding it with the same side arm. Using the opposite hand, grab the inner thigh, taking the thumb and positioning it at the underwear line. You will feel indentations along that line.

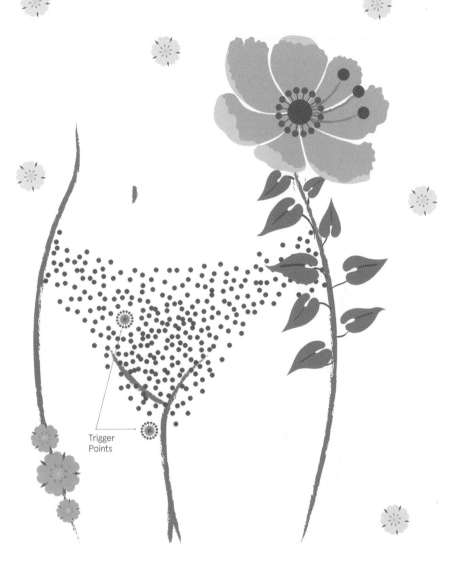

Trigger
Points

Feel into those, and when you find the right spot on your body, press deeply and hold for a count of 30—then move the hand side to side for a count of 30. You might find a lot of other interesting pressure points down there- explore! Then switch sides.

3. The pressure points around the top of the pelvis: the iliac ridge and crest. Get to know the outline of your upper pelvis. Lay on your back. Use your fingertips to find the bony part of the front of your hips. Place your thumbs at the top of that bone, one on each hip, slightly to the inside of the bone, and begin pressing down, walking your thumbs up and around the hip bone, noticing the line and finding the tender spots. When you do find a tender spot, back off slightly, rub it to bring heat, and apply slow pressure to bring blood flow into the area.

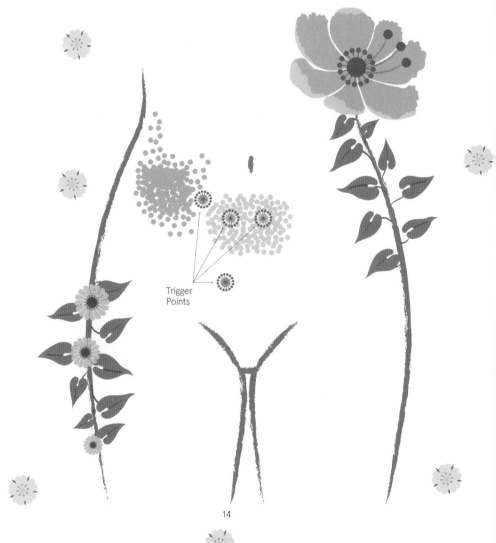

Trigger
Points

4. The pressure points on the sacrum. The sacrum is a hard place to self-massage. One way to do this is to make two fists and reach around your lower back to find the center of your sacrum. Move outward until you find the edge of the bone, where it meets soft tissue. Use your knuckles to make small round motions there. Another technique is to use a tennis ball or other small, firm ball. Lay on your back and place the ball at the edge of the sacrum. Lean into it. Hold for 15 seconds, then reposition the ball and repeat. This is a stronger and deeper method of accessing this important area.

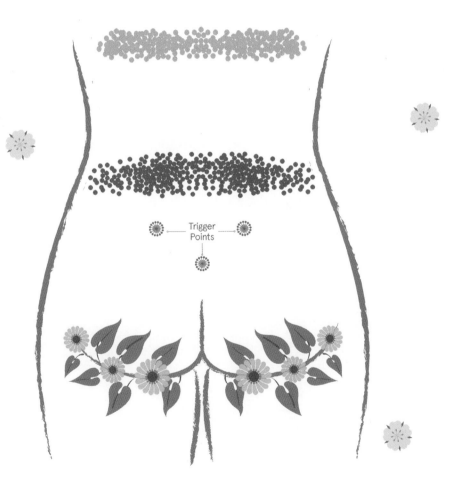

Trigger Points

Strengthening and Opening
the Pelvic Bowl

At the base of the pelvis are intersecting bands of muscles that help to contain the pelvic bowl. This system of muscles can be trained to support full female health, sensuality and sexuality.

Obstetricians, gynecologists, midwives and doulas (birth helpers) often suggest Kegels as an exercise to strengthen the vagina. They say this exercise feels like "stopping the flow of urine." But, stopping urine flow is actually a different muscle set. Once you begin fine tuning your muscular awareness, you will see that the muscles that stop urination, the muscles that allow contraction of the anus, and the muscles that help us engage the vagina are different systems.

A good way to isolate and activate the vaginal and pelvic floor musculature is with what is called "Jade Balls," "Jade Eggs" or "Yoni Eggs." You can look online to find some excellent suggestions for how to practice, what to expect, and how to progressively train the vaginal muscles and get stronger, leading to more sensation and more pleasure.

When you work with the pelvic bowl, you can also begin to open the hip and groin, and the full 360 degree hip and thigh area.

One exercise we really like here is a self adjustment on the pubic bone. Lay on your back, with your knees together and your feet apart, and place two fists between your knees. On the exhale, squeeze the knees as hard as you can together, and hold for 8 counts. Often, you will hear a small pop, and the pubic bone realigns itself.

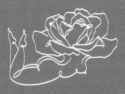

Play in your body. Don't fret about its perceived imperfections. Go out and do stuff, become strong and flexible and free, be naked outside. You are a real thing, you have this one life in this one body. Enjoy it.

The Root Lock

Finally, we want to introduce the Root Lock. In the ancient
Indian practices of yoga, the engagement of this system at
the base of the torso is called the "Root Lock," or in Sanskrit,
"Moola Bandha." It is one of four commonly practiced "locks."
In the image to the right, it begins where the little yellow cross
is located.

The other three locks are at the abdomen, at the chin, and at
the tip of the tongue. When these locks are applied, the spine
and spinal cord are held in such a way as to optimize energy flow.
This improves nervous system communication up and down the
spine, and from the junction boxes on the spine, and out to the
extremities. By connecting the Root Lock to breathing, there
is a sort of gentle pumping mechanism that occurs, which lifts,
strengthens, and oxygenates the pelvic floor.

The original written documentation about Moola Bandha was
done by men, describing their personal experience. What is
different about Moola Bandha in a woman's body?

In the female body, applying the root lock feels different. Our
cavity needs containment. To help with this, we lift UP at the
perineum, as if this intersecting band of muscles was hugging
the tailbone, or as if we were putting a little cap on the tip of
the tailbone. Then, we engage the vaginal cavity and the rectum,
pulling them toward one another (front to back/ back to front),
and finally, we lift the whole system up toward the navel. Our
friend Anna Judd says: "Imagine you had a suppository and a
tampon in at the same time and they were reaching for each
other. That's the action we want to see."

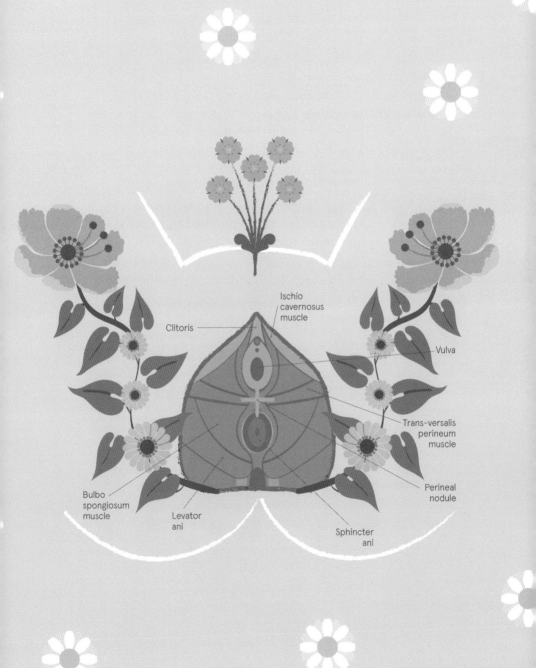

Complex Beauty

There's not a lot of conversation around the complex organs of the general outer genitalia, replete with sensation and opportunities for increased pleasure. Mostly we focus on what is generally (inaccurately) called "the clitoris" because it has so many nerve endings, and ignore all the rest of the parts. This leaves a lot of unexplored territory down there.

MONS PUBIS - Latin for "pubic mound". The mons pubis is the area of skin and subcutaneous fatty tissue that rests on top of the pubic symphysis of the pubic bones, protecting this joint. The mons pubis begins to exhibit hair growth at the onset of puberty, and contains glands that produce pheromones. There are great places along the mons pubis to apply pressure for general tension release. Explore!

Working from outside in, the next thing you will encounter are the LABIA MAJORA– Literally "large lips", this pair of rounded, meaty outer skin folds contains oil and sweat glands. It protects and (sometimes) covers a woman's more delicate inner structures.

As you're looking at your parts, moving from the outer labia inward, you'll notice a place where the skin's texture changes. This is where the skin changes as it meets the more keratinized skin on the labia minora. This is called the HART'S LINE.

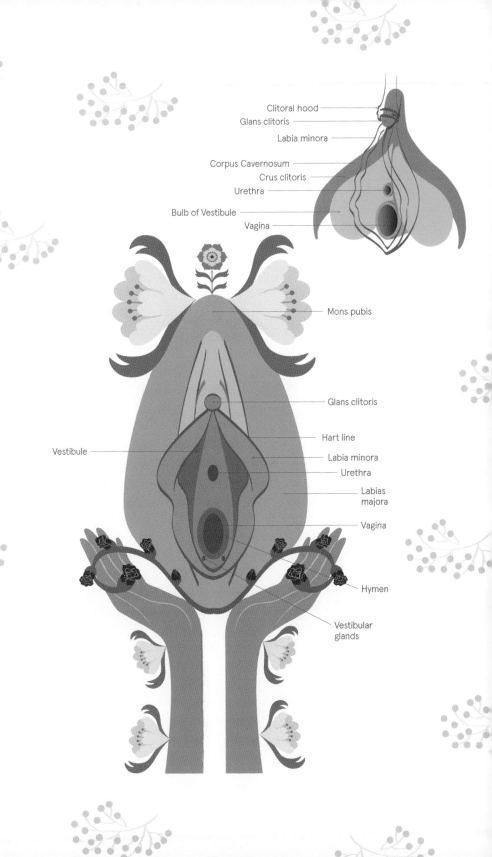

Clitoral hood

Glans clitoris

Labia minora

Corpus Cavernosum

Crus clitoris

Urethra

Bulb of Vestibule

Vagina

Mons pubis

Glans clitoris

Hart line

Vestibule

Labia minora

Urethra

Labias majora

Vagina

Hymen

Vestibular glands

Inside of the labia minora, at the very top, is the CLITORAL HOOD – Also known as the clitoral prepuce, this fold of skin protects and helps maintain sensitivity of the glans clitoris. Interestingly, it is the same kind of tissue as the foreskin, the skin that protects the head of the penis in naturally intact uncircumcised males.

Underneath the hood is the GLANS CLITORIS - Usually, this is what people think of as the clitoris itself. But this button-like external structure is only a small part of the larger hidden system of the clitoris. The size, shape, and color may vary for the glans clitoris, a structure that contains around 8,000 nerve endings vital for arousal and sexual response. It can be barely findable or up to two inches long when engorged.

As you spread the inner lips, open you are in the VESTIBULE – The part of the vulva between the labia minora into which the URETHRA and the vaginal introitus open, you will see the urethral opening - This is where urine exits the body. You will also see the opening to the VAGINA – The elastic muscular tube structure of the female genital tract through which sexual intercourse, childbirth, and menstruation all occur.

As you're exploring, try different kinds of touch, rolling, squeezing and stroking, and note the multitude of sensations on each of these external genitalia, and how they roll out into your body.

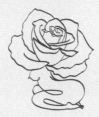

It's common to hear that if you don't love yourself,
you can't love anyone else. The second part, that
you can't receive love from others, is often missed.

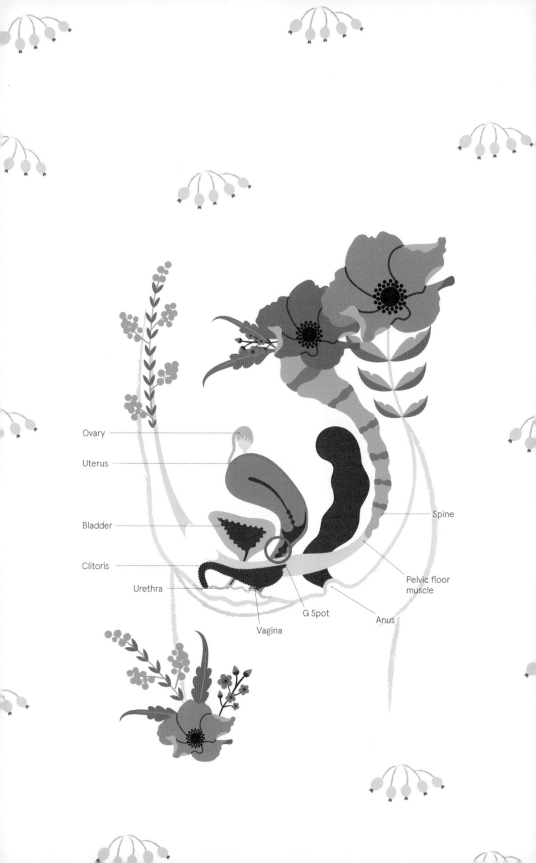

Ovary

Uterus

Bladder

Clitoris

Urethra

Spine

Pelvic floor muscle

Anus

G Spot

Vagina

Secret World: Internal Organs

Once we enter the vaginal canal, we have an entered an entire complex world that is even more often unexplored.

One of the least discussed systems are all of the internal parts of the clitoris. This is a primary locus of female sexual pleasure. It has the shape of a wishbone, and is comprised of erectile tissues, muscles, and nerves. The CRUS CLITORIS – The "crus" (legs) of the clitoris is the pair of internal structures of the clitoris that extends from the corpus cavernosum.

The crus, like all of the erectile tissue of the clitoris, become engorged with blood during arousal. Then come the BULBS OF THE VESTIBULE – These bulbs are an internal part of the clitoris on either side of the vaginal opening, composed of elongated bunches of erectile tissue. And even more broadly, we have the corpus cavernosum – The glans of the clitoris is connected internally to a pair of spongy internal erectile tissues that encompass the vagina on either side, and become erect as they fill with blood during arousal.

The famed "G-SPOT" - or Gräfenberg spot, is a sensitive, spongy bean or dime-shaped area located about 2.5"-5" inches inside the vagina on the upper anterior wall. Some studies suggest the G-spot may be the root of the clitoris. When engorged and stimulated it can produce both powerful orgasms and female ejaculation.

THE VESTIBULAR GLANDS - Found in the vestibule or vagina (Bartholin's and Skene's), these glands secrete mucus to provide vaginal lubrication during sexual arousal.

VAGINA - This elastic muscular tube structure of the female genital tract through which sexual intercourse, childbirth, and menstruation all occur.

HYMEN – Sometimes referred to as the vaginal corona, the hymen is made up of elastic folds of mucous membrane located just inside the vaginal opening (introitus). The hymen does not serve any known function, and may be a vestigial structure from embryological vaginal development.

On the other side of the vagina, through the Cervix, is the uterus – Also called the womb, this hollow upside-down pear shaped organ is made up of three layers of tissue that produces vaginal and uterine secretions. It helps pass male sperm to the fallopian tubes, and hosts any growing fetus.

At the end of the Fallopian tubes are the Ovaries – The two almond-sized primary female reproductive glands that, when mature, are responsible for storing and releasing eggs (oocytes) and the hormones estrogen and progesterone.

Also in this diagram:

PELVIC FLOOR MUSCLE – The pelvic floor is made up of a network of muscles (the levator ani, which are attached to the sacrum and coccygeus), ligaments, and connective tissues. These function like a hammock to support the organs of the pelvis, bladder, cervix, uterus, vagina, and the lower parts of the rectum.

SPINE – The backbone is comprised of a series of bones called vertebrae that extend from the skull to the base of the back and enclose the spinal cord and nerves. It functions as the scaffolding for the entire body, and supports about half the body's weight.

URETHRA – The small transport tube of the renal system that leads urine from the bladder outward during evacuations. Because the female urethra is significantly shorter than the male urethra, females have a higher risk of developing urinary tract infections.

BLADDER – Located at the base of the pelvis, this muscular organ functions as a reservoir that can expand like a balloon to hold 1.5-2 cups of urine, which empty through the urethra.

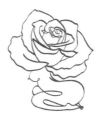

There was a moment when she realized no one was coming to save her. She had allies, but her life was on her. This was the first step to freedom.

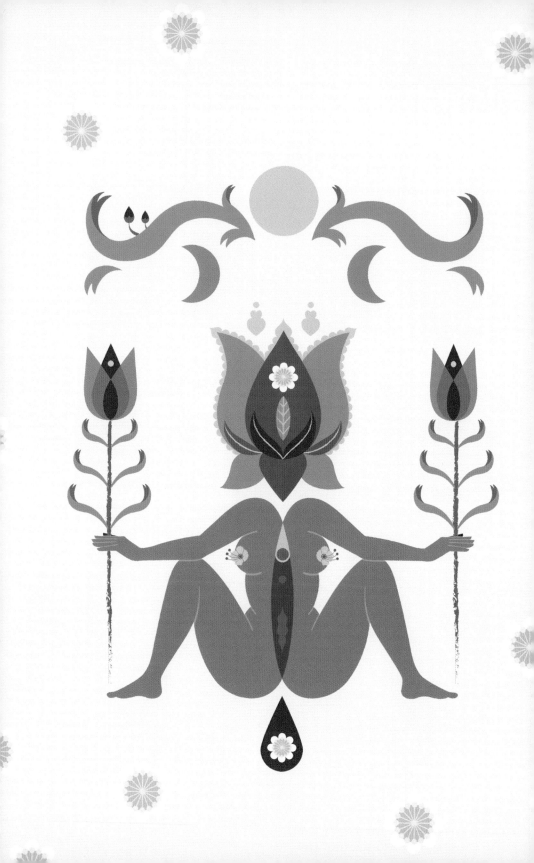

Part 3: Life in Cycles

A woman's physical life (when honored and intact) is cyclical and in harmony with nature. She runs on the schedule of the moon and seasons. In all of her cycles there is a building, a cresting, a fading, and a stillness. This holds true for her life's reproductive cycle, her monthly reproductive cycle, the wave and crest of her sexual experience, the wave and crest of her bearing, and the alignment of her body with seasonal cycles.

The dominant culture of assembly lines, clock time, and digitized life often overrides natural rhythms, and can interfere with these cycles. You know that the condition of your skin is not the same, depending on where you are in your cycles—but our product-based manufacturing culture, run on a more linear assumption base, will treat you as static. It's easier to make and sell things to meet a static need. A cyclical life is more subtle, and has more nuance.

Those of us who have jobs and families and live and love in the material world can't exactly run our lives on our personal cycles. But we can make minor adjustments that tune us in more closely with the underlying reality of these cycles. We might make the first day or two of our moon time less active and more introspective, taking some extra time for self-care on those days. We might make our peak fertility days of the month the deliberate time for being out in the world, playing and adventuring. We might relearn the traditional stages of the female life, from girl (prepubescent), to maiden (pubescent but not a mother), to woman (potentially a mother) to matron (when the last child is grown, or a woman has gone through menopause) and create graduations honoring these passages in ourselves and others. Many cultures mark these milestones, but not many people in the west do this in an intentional way.

The thing about not marking such milestones in a community of women is, we don't know what's "normal." You'll see a lot of "averages" thrown out in women's health- such as "the average age of menarche is 12.8," or, "the average age of menopause is 52." However, these disguise the wild fluctuations in the distribution curve. For example, breast buds in girls can start as early as eight, and as late as 14. The first period arrives as early as nine and as late as 15. First menopause symptoms can start at a wild variation of ages- from 40 to 65. 35% of women experience their symptom onsets between 50 and 54. Sources might tell you that a menstrual cycle is 28 days long- but it can range from 21 to 45 days. You might hear a normal pregnancy is 40 weeks- but anything from 38 to 42 weeks is considered normal.

Find your own rhythm, your own normal. Self love means, in part, overriding the dominant culture and taking care of yourself, and attuning to your own personal biology.

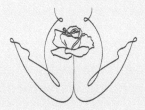

When we love our whole being, and know our worth, self-love
inevitably becomes Self-love, with a capital S. We are made of the
same energy as all creation, and are never separate.

Part 4: Looking Inside Yourself

If you've lived your life based primarily on responses to external approval, or with strong personalities surrounding and influencing you, you may have lost all sense of who you are: what you actually feel, sense, and think inside. Personal development teacher Thomas Huebl says that this state creates an inner fragmentation and splitting. When this lack of wholeness is the norm, the scattered state of our nervous system seems like our "normal" state.

So how do we relearn how to look and listen inward?

Dr. Cat Meyer, a psychotherapist and yoga therapist, says that one of the first movements she makes with her clients is to "introcept": to look inward as an antidote to objectification, to taking in and being quantified by the outside world: "What's real for me? What's inside of my own experience?"

Thomas Huebl speaks of this as well. He calls it "looking in silence." No entertainment, nothing from outside, is needed. The importance of simple presence—the ability to know what we feel, and be completely present with ourselves, and our experience—can't be underestimated.

This doesn't mean it's easy. A lot of feelings come up when you're beginning to relax around places that have hardened in memory, belief, body. "When you're in a stage where there is heating and stuff is melting," Huebl continues, "you're being more sensitive, and the emotional heat feels like it's getting stronger." What to do? Jacques Verduin, a Buddhist teacher, calls the development of the spaciousness inside to deal with these feelings "Sitting in the Fire." Looking at the hurt or fear we carry, and staying with the discomfort as it builds and then dissolves- until we come out the other side clear and clean.

Conversely, you might not feel anything in the beginning stages of this "inner melting." Sometimes you've over-regulated your own insides, and just feel numb. But "even if you feel numbness," Huebl says, "just let the numbness be. Look inside with your numbness and fear, including it in your experience. Even if you don't know where to look! Just keep looking."

I personally practice vipassana meditation, which includes sitting in silence for long periods of time. Silence gives me the spaciousness to deal with what Huebl calls "the incongruence in my nervous system" and to tell the difference between my pre-existing filters and what is real, here, now, actual, and accurate.

This "inner precision" needs practice.

But if you try this technique you might find, as I did, that the relational structure you have with your inner life mirrors the relational structure you present with other people. An inner life of presence, ease and self love and care ripples out into the world. Teacher Laura Plumb says "Self-care is World-care." And that makes you a present powerful being in whatever you do.

You can practice being present and spacious in many ways: being in nature, alone with yourself, for an hour or more, and practicing looking inside yourself and noticing what you actually feel and think; trying different styles of meditation practice until you find one that takes you into a more open, expansive quality of mind; participating in a retreat or program with a great teacher in person or online. All of these things help you be in a space where all you do is focus on your sensory and inner experience. It's worth the investment in living your life. Self-love and self-care begin within.

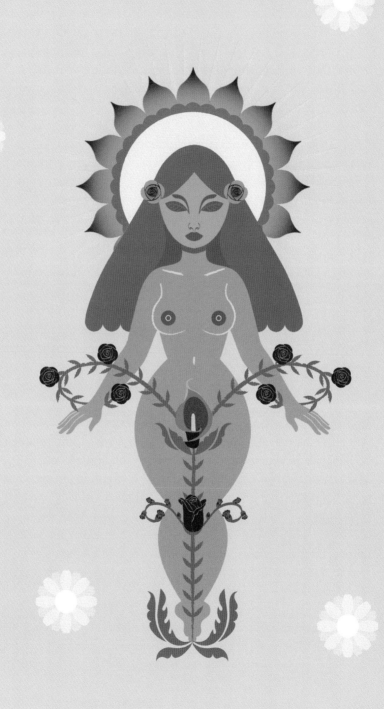

Part 5: The Journey into Conscious Sensuality

(rewritten and adapted from Robert Silber on Conscious Sensuality)

Conscious sensuality is all about widening the range of what's possible. The journey into conscious sensuality prioritizes the importance and value of sensations and emotions in our lives. In this practice, we affirm that experiencing and expressing our sensations and emotions to the world around us is valuable, and that it matters. This helps us feel more in our bodies, or be "embodied." It helps us to experience emotions more deeply.

Doing this also develops our capacity to choose how to respond to our emotions. This is a crucial distinction, as just having strong emotions and strong reactions does not indicate a balanced emotional body. To develop our consciousness, we must place primary emphasis on awareness of our own sensations and emotions. When we have limited emotional and sensory ranges, we often substitute thought for emotion and sensation. When we are too caught up in our minds, our lives are out of balance and we are unhealthy.

SENSUALITY ISN'T THE SAME AS SEXUALITY

Sexual repression can make us see everything sensual as sexual. Most people link sensuality and sexuality so closely in their minds that it prevents their sensual awareness and enjoyment. While people may confuse the two, sensual refers to all the senses, not just physical touch and the activation of sensors on our skin.Sensual includes the enjoyment of all of our senses of taste, touch, sight, hearing, and smell. It is true that all of the senses can play a part in sexual excitement and sexual connection. But can we enjoy a hug or a back rub that has no sexual energy behind it? Can we hear beautiful music and feel transported to a place of peace and tranquility? Our senses give us gifts of pleasure, and opportunities for greater awareness.

Imagine life with no senses at all. We would hardly seem alive. Yet mind would remain. In fact, sensory deprivation is a key practice that can assist the consciousness raising experiences. Sitting in meditation is a form of sensory deprivation that allows us to develop mindfulness: a perspective where we are more conscious of the mind. Sitting in silent meditation is a key practice for building awareness, and can be useful in resetting the emotional body.

By intentionally isolating the senses we can increase our capacity for sensual experience. Blocking out one sense often heightens the perception of other senses, which is why the blind often excel at music, or even touch. In Thailand, for example, massage is a natural profession for the blind.

WORKING WITH YOUR EMOTIONAL BODY

Good sexual connection is the fruit of health, joy, and connection to oneself, not a strategy to cope with loneliness, fear of inadequacy, or emotional release through cathartic orgasms.

KNOW THYSELF

Before we get to sexual excitement with a lover, we might first focus on generating our own natural energy through yoga, meditation, nourishing food, sleep, and release of emotional charges. Our task is to first work on ourselves, and get to know our own terrain. Which means we must come to understand our conditioned or learned reactions to different types of stimulation: to learn what we like and what we dislike, to distinguish between our desires and our addictions, to love ourselves even when we are very disappointed, and to love others even when we do not understand them.

One of the first steps is to make an accurate assessment of what we want, why we think we want it (is it a goal, or a strategy to get to something else?), and to release all that is in the way of receiving love and connection.

This can be the scariest part of coming into consciousness. To be honest with others is to first be honest with ourselves— and in the process we may appear less attractive to others. In essence, we need to clean house before filling ourselves up with someone else's concepts and techniques. Once the space is empty, let us not rush to fill it up, but rather selectively integrate what resonates at a deep level and learn to be at peace with not having all the answers. We need not have a completely integrated psycho-spiritual-sexual-intellectual framework to have connection and love in our lives—but we do need honesty, curiosity, and courage.

GIVE YOURSELF EMPATHY

When we release our own emotions in a safe way, we can be available to understand and connect with others. Rather than shaming, blaming, and giving "shoulds" to others, we can acknowledge what emotions we experience and what we want. Releasing emotions is easier when we receive empathy: the presence of a loving witness who feels with us. This could be a friend. Counselors, coaches or therapists can also be of incredible value here. They don't absorb our emotions or stories about others, and won't argue or block the release of our emotions.

Ultimately, it is essential that we learn how to give ourselves empathy and clear our emotional body by ourselves, but this is an advanced practice. At the beginning of your journey it is crucial to seek out empathy from others to learn the processes and break through your walls of fear, shame, and self-judgment.

IF YOU'RE SHUT DOWN...

When working within the realm of sexuality, the emotions are so intense, and the sensations so acute, that we can easily shut down or become overwhelmed. Shutting down or getting overloaded happens when we have emotions that exceed our ability to assimilate and express them consciously. To move past emotional numbness or dysfunctional emotional reactivity that pushes others away, we must increase our emotional range and our awareness about what exactly we are experiencing. If this is you, be patient. Know that you came by your shut down honestly, that it served you at some point in your life. Start where you are, go slow.

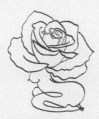

In the great sisterhood, we celebrate each other's
successes, as if it were happening to us.
On a deeper level, it is anyway.

Part 6: Touch and Self Massage

THE IMPORTANCE OF TOUCH

Touch is the the first sense to develop in babies,and with good reason. Touch is literally life or death for an infant. The amount of touch sets a baby's metabolism. Babies deprived of touch have a stunted metabolism, and don't grow correctly.

In nonhuman primates, touch is a vital part of their cooperative social compact: They spend between 10% and 20% of each day grooming each other. As adult humans, most of us don't get enough of this!

IN ADULTS, TOUCH:

·   calms cardiovascular stress
·   boosts the immune system
·   stimulates the part of the brain necessary for memory
·   releases healthy hormones
    (including Oxytocin, the "love and trust" hormone)
·   lowers cortisol (the stress hormone)
·   enhances metabolic functioning
·   stimulates lymph function

Touch is also called the primary language of compassion. It makes people feel more connected, cooperative, and less threatened. Musician Mary Chapin Carpenter says it so beautifully:

We all hit the ground, we all fall from the sky
We burn up, we break up, we wreck and we cry
But we're bound up together by sight and by pact
That begins with the touch of your hand on my back

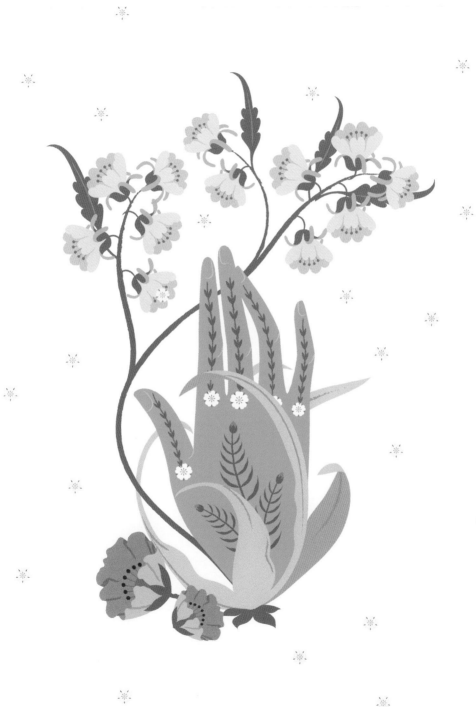

Dacher Keltsen's lab (as cited in the professional journal Emotion) has discovered some unexpected benefits of touch: Professional basketball teams, for example, win more games if the players touch each other more.

TOUCH: THE BASICS

Ideally, all the tissues of the body have good blood flow, solid lymphatic circulation, muscular strength, stability, softness, suppleness, and appropriate fluidity. We are also looking for an absence of pain and inflammation. Touch can help with this.

Touch has three main aspects: Location, Speed, and Pressure. By referring to touch in this way, we build a language that allows the giver and receiver to communicate more accurately and thus create more pleasure.

By using this precise language, we empower ourselves to ask for exactly what we want. And by being clear we help the giver to relax into their sensations and emotions, confident that they are giving us touch that is enjoyable.

It is a simple way to practice touch—unlike massage theory, where one needs to remember anatomical names and massage strokes. Many people who have never even taken a massage class have an intuitive sense of what feels good.

SELF-MASSAGE EXERCISES AND RITUALS

1. THE POWER SPOT EXERCISE

The Power Spots are: the feet, the genitals, the belly, the middle of the chest, the third-eye point (a little bit above the point between the eyebrows), the top of the head, the occipital ridge at the base of the skull and the top of the neck, and the sacrum. All of these places have the potential to awaken strong emotions and memories. It is useful to remember that the point of this exercise to access these strong emotions and memories.This is not a massage, so there is no movement, nor a change in pressure—just solid, consistent touch that brings energy and awareness to this part of the body.

If it's comfortable for you to sit cross legged, and begin with your feet, do so. Alternating feet, feel around until you find a sensitive or responsive spot, or pressure point. Apply pressure with the thumb and the whole hand, hold, and don't move the hands again until you lift off and disengage from this power spot.

Progress through each of the power spots. The sacrum will be difficult to reach yourself with a lot of pressure, so a gentle placement of your hands on your hips, getting as close to the sacrum as you can, will do. Hold and release.

By going slowly, paying attention and encouraging activation of the emotional body, we provide an opportunity to access and release whatever is keeping us from being in the present moment and being in our natural state of joy.
This is a wonderful exercise to do with a friend- for both giver and receiver.

2. THE AIRBRUSHING RITUAL

The Airbrushing Ritual is focused on using extremely light touch to sensitize or resensitize the body, and to access the emotional body and whatever blocks may exist. It's almost a tickle or a caress.

This exercise is best done without any clothing on. The point is to find where your blocks are, and create an opportunity to bring to consciousness any emotions that are inhibiting the natural flow of energy. The airbrushing ritual should be done energetically at first, and then skin to skin as lightly as possible. You can vary the speed, and move between light touch and no touch—but do not go into deeper touch or start to massage specific parts of the body. In this way, the whole body is energized, awakened, and expanded.

3. KEEPING TWO OF THREE CONSTANT EXERCISE

Work with any parts of your body that are calling to you: think thighs, forearms, hands, face. Leave nothing out.

By altering each of the three individual aspects of touch— location, speed, and pressure—while maintaining consistency with the other two, you can focus on exactly the most pleasurable point of the range of that particular aspect. For example, you might want to explore varying the speed of your touch. Keep the location and pressure the same. Just vary the speed from slow to very fast, and every speed in between. Next, try changing the pressure, while keeping the speed and location the same... and so on.

4.   THE SELF-PLEASURING RITUAL

Give yourself at least 1/2 hour or more for this ritual. The idea is to massage ourselves all over our bodies, and to give ourselves the touch we would like to receive from another person. Though women are culturally sanctioned to nurture themselves, all the beautification, pampering, spa treatments, etc., are often part of a strategy to please men and society, rather than for self-care or self-love purposes. Use a good massage oil, such as almond or coconut oil. Using oil helps to warm up and loosen the body; it increases fluidity in the strokes, which encourages relaxation.

SET THE TONE:

Start with a prayer, an intention, and some deep breathing to center yourself. Turn on some slow meditative music, which will help you relax and go slowly. Create the space around you to reflect how you would like things to be on this very special date: a date with yourself.

BREASTS, SHOULDER AND UPPER ARMS:

Begin touching yourself by placing one hand on your belly, and the other between your breasts at the heart center. Move the hand that's on the heart up and across the breast to the shoulder, down the upper arm and then back up under the breast. Switch hands as you come through the center point, and go to the other side. It will essentially be a figure eight, accessing the muscles of the chest and shoulder and rib cage and torso. If you like, you can give special attention to your nipples, generating more erotic energy in your system.

HEAD, FACE AND NECK:

Anywhere the bones of the skull give way to cartilage or muscle, there can be tension. Try connecting with your jaw, nose bridge, cheekbones, eye sockets and forehead, and the hairline. Give loving attention to areas such as your eyes and ears. Try pulling, twisting, and gently touching your ears, encouraging them to release stored tension. Go to the top of your head and massage along the big jaw muscles that attach to the peak of the crown, and drift back to the ridge where the spine and the skull come together.

Move down your neck onto your chest and give yourself a firm massage, stretching the powerful muscles in your chest.

BELLY, LOWER BACK, BUTTOCKS, LEGS AND FEET:

Now move towards your belly, and massage your stomach and other internal organs. Moving your hands in the direction of digestion from the right to the left side of your belly and down towards the pelvic region. Now massage your lower back, contacting the sacrum and your kidneys. Moving down, massage your buttocks, then down each of your legs towards your feet. Give special attention to your feet. You can spend a long time massaging someone else's feet—why not your own?

GENITALS:

Having given loving attention to every area of your body except your genitals, you are now ready to give them some attention as well. Maintain the same loving attention and touch that you just gave to the rest of your body. See if you can massage yourself in a slow, pleasurable way, without needing to orgasm or ejaculate. See if you can be present to the sensation in your body without going into fantasy.

When you feel complete, whether you have had an orgasm or not, return to a place of stillness with a hand on the heart and one on your genitals. Stay with you your breath for a few minutes as you absorb the energy of this experience. Witness your thoughts, emotions, and sensations.

5. FOCUS: CHEST, HEART, AND BREAST TOUCH RITUAL

The first stage of breast touch involves holding one's hand over the heart or the center of the chest. This can even be done without making contact, but by just holding a hand a few inches away. Or, if desired, the hand can be placed with medium light stationary pressure over the center of the chest. Just holding a hand here can be enough to encourage relaxation and major emotional release.

The second stage of breast touch is to massage the breasts without contacting the nipple area, which is more sensitive and erotically charged. One of the best and more important strokes is to hold the arm over the head and massage down the arm, over the armpit and down the side of the breast towards the feet. This helps drain the fluid from the lymph nodes in this region. This is where breast cancer often starts. (Note: It is recommended that women do self-examination of their breasts on a regular basis. Considering that breast cancer is a leading cause of death for middle-aged women, it is imperative that we demystify and encourage breast touch.)

Lymphatic drainage strokes can come very close to the nipples without touching them, or remain further away. Either way, with this long, even stroke, the breast is connected and integrated with the rest of the body.

You can then massage around the whole breast and the nipples. At first you may want to just slide over the nipples, which wakes up the nerve receptors and integrates the nipples with the breasts and the rest of the body. If desired, you can give special attention to the nipples by lightly grazing, then squeezing, rolling, and pulling them.

This may build up erotic energy. After a while of breast and nipple massage, simply move away and towards another area of the body. It greatly helps to expand the range of sensation and response if you do not move directly from your breasts to your genitals. One way to re-pattern sexuality is by changing the standard sequence of breast touch followed immediately by genital touch. This also allows for the energy generated in the breasts to be spread and integrated into the rest of the body.

6. FOCUS: CONSCIOUS GENITAL TOUCH

Conscious genital touch is a way of un-patterning our sexual conditioning, and releasing us from goal-oriented sexual behavior. We can just lie down and touch ourselves, or be touched, without needing to do anything else. This is very relaxing—though it can be challenging to someone whose pattern is to give, or who has a fear of receiving from another.

This is a time to slow down, breathe, open, and connect with oneself without any goal. This is a meditative practice. Just like sitting in meditation—a non-sexual form of meditation—it can greatly increase our consciousness by allowing us to watch the mind.

This act of witnessing, or mindfulness, cultivates sensitivity, which is an important part of building connection with others and ourselves. To be sensitive to our bodies and our emotions is to increase our capacity to know ourselves. And by increasing that capacity to know ourselves, we increase our knowing of others. We can only be as perceptive with others as we are with ourselves.

1. EXTERIOR MASSAGE

    Start by massaging the pubic mound and then the outer labia. Massaging slowly from the outside towards the midline and opening of the vagina. Take plenty of time to massage up and down, focusing on making contact with every area repeatedly and connecting all the areas together in long slow strokes. Try not to dissociate: stay present with yourself.

2. CONNECTING WITH THE GLANS CLITORIS

    After massaging the pubic mound and the outer and inner labia, move on to contacting the clitoris. This bundle of nerves and tissues comes to head above the introitus, or opening of the vagina. Some women have a pronounced clitoral hood that can obscure the clitoris entirely, or barely at all. The clitoral nerves extend from the clitoris down either side of the external genitalia, beneath the labia. This means that when we are massaging up and down the labia we are already starting to make contact with the clitoris, which prepares the clitoris for more direct contact. The root of the clitoris is the famed G spot, so in touching this we are also lighting the inner fire.

    It may feel best to make contact with and massage

over the hood of the clit first, before pulling the hood back and making directly contact with the clitoris. It's important to note that, if you have a pronounced clitoral hood that completely covers the clitoris, you may have difficulty pulling the hood back. This can be especially true if you have used too much lubricant.

The point of massaging the clitoris is not just for stimulation or orgasm, but to connect it with the rest of the vagina, and to use the energy generated by clitoral stimulation to make internal vagina touch desired. Some people perform self-massage sessions without focusing on the clitoris, because it can be very arousing and thus distract from the other parts of the body and the yoni. One good approach is to contact the clitoris, but not to give it too much attention—just enough attention to put energy in the system

3. PULSING AT THE VESTIBULE

An often overlooked area of the pussy is the vestibule or the introitus. It's useful to pay attention to this gatekeeper. During sex, this area is often overlooked in the hurry to penetrate the vagina. If the woman is not sufficiently aroused and lubricated, this area can be stressed or even torn in the mad rush to get inside. There are a lot of nerves in this area, and massaging it can be very pleasurable.

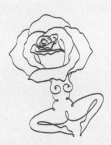

Life operates in waves: the ocean, music, life cycles,
pregnancies, even orgasms. To enter, build, explode,
resolve and return to stillness.
- GABRIELLE ROTH

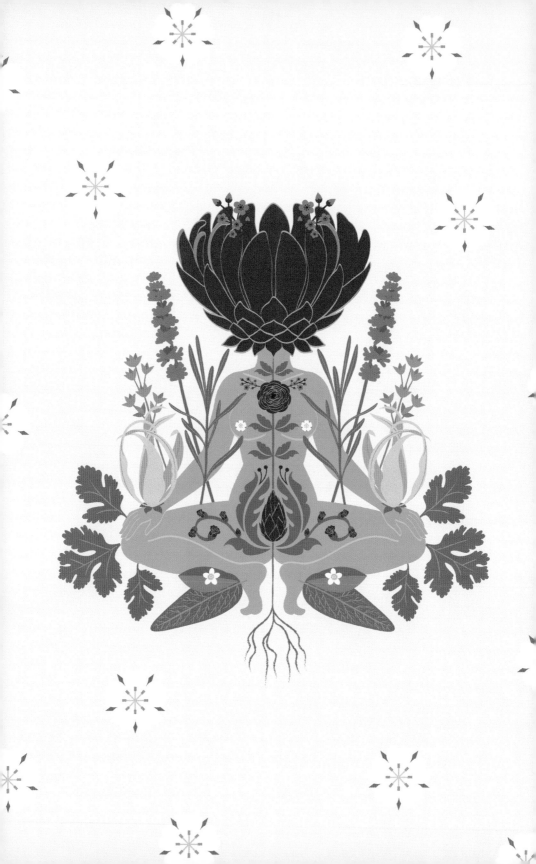

Part 7: Lowering the "Body Load"

During the last 70 years, we have been running a massive experiment on our bodies. This dates from the onset of packaged foods, plastics, polyester clothing, treated upholstery, cleaning supplies, fertilizers, and pesticides. We don't yet know the long term effects. We do know however, that traces of all of these things show up in our skin and eyes and gut biomes and... well, everywhere in the body.

Even naturally occuring substances, such as minerals from the earth, used to be released slowly into the environment through various natural processes. Minerals are released at a steady pace through the wearing away of rock by erosion (which puts minerals into the atmosphere through the water cycle) as well as periodic volcanic eruptions, which send particles high into the air. Today, minerals are mined and spewed into the atmosphere and into our products at toxic levels.

The organs that clean the blood are taking it hard: The liver (which processes parts of our food) and the kidneys (the organs that process waste and toxins) are showing increased incidents of cancers. Liver cancer is now the most rapidly increasing cause of cancer death in the U.S.. Incidence of liver cancer began rising in the mid-1970s, while the rate of new kidney cancers has been rising since the 1990s. For men, sperm count is plummeting worldwide, largely ascribed to environmental toxins such as estrogen-inducing phthalates in plastics.

The amount of toxins that your body has to deal with comprise the "body load." We want to reduce this load anywhere possible, for the sake of our overall health. While it may seem overwhelming to try to combat all the harmful environmental factors that surround us, it is possible to mitigate them and to minimize our exposure in the first place.

Perhaps the most direct way to approach this challenge is by looking at what we put in our bodies and call "food." It is of course preferable to eat fresh, organic, non-GMO foods that are as locally sourced as possible—this aids the body's ability to handle outside stressors, and perform optimally. According to a survey about detoxification therapies published in the Journal of Alternative and Complementary Medicine, 75% of licensed naturopathic doctors, "included dietary measures (cleansing foods, increased fruit/vegetable intake, vitamin/mineral/antioxidant supplementation, organic foods, elimination diet, stool bulking agents/fiber), probiotics, reducing environmental exposure, and cholagogue herbs (herbs that promote the excretion of bile)."

One easy trick to help with this is to shop at the perimeter of grocery stores—where the fresh food is usually displayed—and venture into the aisles of processed food in boxes, bags, and cans only when necessary. Purging the fridge of potentially harmful consumables is one good step.

The next step is to nix the non-stick cookware, plastic wrap, plastic containers and aluminum foil. Stop drinking out of plastic bottles and eating out of Styrofoam boxes. Use natural cleaning products (no propylene glycol, parabens, petroleum, PEGs, and SLS). Then, examine the ingredients on your personal care products. According to a survey by the Environmental Working Group, the average woman uses 12 products containing 168 unique ingredients every day, some of them probable human carcinogens (men use an average of six products daily with 85 unique ingredients).

In these findings it was revealed that "one of every five adults is potentially exposed every day to all of the top seven carcinogenic impurities common to personal care product ingredients — hydroquinone, ethylene dioxide, 1,4-dioxane, formaldehyde, nitrosamines, PAHs, and acrylamide.

The top most common impurity ranked by number of people exposed is hydroquinone, which is a potential contaminant in products used daily by 94 percent of all women and 69 percent of all men."

It's high time to empty our bathroom cabinets, makeup bags and shower caddies, all rife with bioaccumulative toxins!

But the very best way to approach detoxification is through what we do for ourselves on a daily basis. Here are the basics:

EAT CLEAN.

Eat a varied diet full of plenty of organically grown fresh fruits and vegetables—especially foods high in fiber.

WATER.

Drink at least two quarts of water a day, and be aware of where your water is sourced and how much fluoride it contains (some studies have linked fluoride to neurotoxicity and brain damage).

EXERCISE.

Yoga, brisk walking, jump rope, rebounding... it doesn't have to be a boot camp style regimen, but get out there and move for an hour each day. The lymphatic system, which collects and moves waste in the blood, is the only system in the body without a pump—putting the body through daily physical movement is critical, and aids in detoxification.

DRY BRUSH YOUR ENTIRE BODY.

Skin is the largest organ, and the practice of dry brushing can stimulate the lymphatic system, improve circulation, aid exfoliation, and help your skin tone and texture become more even and glowing. Start from the feet and work up toward the heart—long strokes over the long bones, and circular motions around the joints (take care not to be too rough on the abdomen or breasts).

COLD SHOWERS.

Hydrotherapy using cold showers (except during menstruation, or if there are blood pressure problems). The practice of standing under bracing cold water for a few minutes helps clean the circulatory system, strengthens the sympathetic and parasympathetic nervous systems, helps balance glands, brings blood to the capillaries, and keeps the skin vibrant. Alternating between saunas or warm water and ice cold blasts can aid the vasoconstriction/vasodilation process, and boost the benefits of this simple (and cost-effective) practice.

BREATHE.

When we are stressed, we tend to hold our breath. By becoming conscious of our breath, and maintaining regular and easeful inhales and exhales, we can allow oxygen to move more freely through our bodies. One of the six yogic cleansing techniques is Kapalbhati, or "skull-shining breath." This is practiced by sitting comfortably, breathing in through both nostrils, and then—with a sharp exhale— contracting the abdominal muscles toward the spine and pulling up slightly toward the diaphragm. Allow the inhale to come passively and then repeat, always pumping the belly with the exhale for 3-4 sets of 10 'pumps'. (Note: This detoxifying and tonifying pranayama yoga practice is contraindicated for pregnancy, high blood pressure, GERD, heart disease, or abdominal surgeries/pain.)

In Ayurveda, the South Asian "Science of Life", it is considered that one of the root causes of disease is "a crime against wisdom"—in other words, acting against our better instincts and common sense. This happens whenever we go against our internal voice that wants us to care for our body-mind-spirit. It can show up as getting too little sleep, poor nutrition choices and/or overeating, not heeding the body's natural signals to eliminate, binge watching TV (or overusing mobile devices), overindulging in sexual activity, smoking cigarettes, drinking in excess, doing drugs, using products that are toxic, holding on to harmful emotions, etc.

We know deep down what is right and good for our bodies, yet we ignore these inner convictions and thus create opportunity for imbalance and disease to take hold. Adherence to a daily routine that is optimized for our body's constitutional makeup is one way for us to remain aligned with the cosmic wisdom that flows within each of us. When we reclaim control over our lives and pay attention to how we treat ourselves on a daily basis, we rely less and less on diet gurus and medical doctors to tell us what to do, or how to fix ourselves.

This is real self-love!

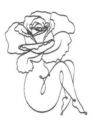

Fall back, my lovely, and be held by the sunshine
and the air and the earth itself, which are always
supporting you.

Part 8: Caring for the Skin and Tissues

UNDERSTANDING THE SKIN YOU'RE IN.

As Harvard Health says, "You may routinely pamper your face and work hard to keep it moisturized and irritation-free—but what have you done lately for the more sensitive skin of your vulva, the external genital area surrounding your vagina?"

The tissues of the vagina are made up of many layers of distinct epithelium called 'strata.' And just like the body's skin (the epidermis), the vaginal epithelium is differentiated into three layers: a bottom (basal) layer, a middle layer (super basal), and a top or superficial layer (the stratum corneum or 'horny layer'). This top layer is made up of of a flattened layer of cells that have filled with a protein called keratin. These topmost, keratinized cells are what make our skin generally waterproof and resilient.

The skin of the vulva is more permeable than other tissues. Here's why.

Knowing about how these cells function helps explain why the tissues of the vagina are more permeable than any other skin on the body (other than the mouth). Non-keratinized epithelium are generally more permeable to external substances. The vulva, just like oral tissue, has different structures and less keratinization that other kinds of skin. The skin of the vulva is ten times more permeable to water alone than is keratinized skin!

The vagina usually maintains a certain minimum moisture level of about 1 milliliter of secretions. These come from sources in the follicles, tubes, uterus, cervix, vagina, and Bartholin and Skene's glands. It is important to note that the skin itself has no glands, so there is no mucus secretion.

This base-level moisture is usually not enough lubrication for any vaginal penetration to be painless.

Right below the three layers of the epithelium is a layer of connective tissue. It is filled with many elastic fibers and blood vessels that assist the exchange of fluid. This layer is essentially a pump that helps the epithelium release and re-absorb just the right amount of fluid through the epithelium. When blood flow increases in an area, the blood vessels in this layer get swollen, and they apply pressure to squeeze and push more water through the epithelium. This fluid is mixed with cervical mucus, and the combination provides lubrication during sexual arousal and intercourse. As arousal increases, droplets of this viscous fluid join to form a slippery layer on the vaginal epithelium. This slightly decreases the acidity of the fluid that's already present. Triggered by neural responses during arousal, the blood supply to the vaginal epithelium increases—but veins drain away the blood more slowly, causing engorgement. This enhances the permeability of the tissues even further.

Moreover, the vaginal skin is impacted by hormones and environmental factors during a woman's lifespan, as well as during each of our menstrual cycles and menopause. A healthy vaginal epithelium usually can fight off infections and sexually transmitted diseases. During ovulation, glycogen stored in the vaginal epithelium peaks. Later, as it breaks down, it produces lactic acid. This shifts the pH of the vagina to more acidic levels that stop the growth of bacteria, fungus, and other pathogens—but also make it tougher for any sperm present to survive.

Understanding the sensitivity and permeability of the vaginal skin leads many of us to examine and question the ingredients used in many personal care products, and seek alternate products that are natural and plant-based.

To protect your pussy, here are some common ingredients to avoid:

Parabens, according to the Environmental Working Group, "are a class of chemicals used as preservatives in food, industrial products and personal care products, but most widely prevalent in cosmetics and personal care products." Nearly everyone is exposed to these compounds: The U.S. Centers for Disease Control and Prevention tested more than 2,500 urine samples, and detected methyl paraben in 99 percent and propyl paraben in 93 percent.

Although parabens are "generally recognized as safe" in foods by the U.S. Food and Drug Administration, increasing evidence has drawn attention to their possible health risks— primarily their potential to disrupt the endocrine system, which can interfere with the normal functioning of hormones. This, in turn, may potentially switch on the growth of hormone-receptor-positive breast cancers.

Propylene glycol is a liquid solvent used as an antifreeze as well as to absorb excess water or maintain moisture in certain medicines, cosmetics, and food products. Also classified as "generally recognized as safe" by the U.S. Food and Drug Administration it is a known allergen for some. It is possibly toxic to kidneys and the liver, and exposure may be linked to heart disease. Its use is potentially even more risky for highly permeable areas of the body—like the vaginal epithelium— because of its excellent ability to increase the penetration and absorption of accompanying substances and chemicals.

Petrochemicals prevent normal cell and skin functions when applied topically, and present a host of threatening issues. Petroleum products produce 1,4-dioxane, which causes cancer and is also toxic to the kidneys, nervous system, and respiratory system. When possible, avoid:

- MINERAL OIL

- ANYTHING WITH PEG (POLYETHYLENE GLYCOL)

- ANYTHING ENDING IN 'ETH' indicates that it required ethylene oxide (a petrochemical) to produce e.g. myreth, oleth, laureth, ceteareth

- ANYTHING WITH DEA (diethanolamine) or MEA (ethanolamine)

- BUTANOL AND ANY WORD WITH 'BUTYL' – butyl alcohol, butylparaben, butylene glycol

- ETHANOL AND WORD WITH 'ETHYL' – ethyl alcohol, ethylene glycol, ethylene dichloride, EDTA (ethylene-diamine-tetracetatic acid), ethylhexylglycerin

- ANY WORD WITH "PROPYL" – isopropyl alcohol, propylene glycol, propyl alcohol, cocamidopropyl betaine

- METHANOL AND ANY WORD WITH 'METHYL' – methyl alcohol, methylparaben, methylcellulose

- TOLUENE

- BENZENE

- PHENOXYETHANOL

- PARAFFIN WAX

- The general terms "PARFUM" or "FRAGRANCE" – 95% of chemicals used in fragrance are from petroleum.

- Silicone oils such as DIMETHICONE, etc. Similar to petroleum by-products they coat and smother the skin, and are potentially an irritant and toxin.

- PHTHALATES, According to the Environmental Working Group, "are a widely used group of endocrine-disrupting chemicals that have been linked to problems of the reproductive system, including hormonal changes, thyroid irregularities and birth defects in the reproductive systems of baby boys. Used as a plasticizer, they are ubiquitous in household products such as food containers, children's toys, plastic wrap made from polyvinyl chloride (PVC) as well as many cosmetics and personal care products. In cosmetics, phthalates are typically used to maintain the scent of fragrances in many colognes, perfumes, hair products, deodorants, lotions, body washes and much more."

THE GOOD STUFF: Treat your lady bits right with these natural aids for lubrication, moisture, and blood flow.

- NATURAL OILS provide a much safer solution to aiding vaginal lubrication. Organic ghee (clarified butter), coconut, sesame, grapeseed, olive, sweet almond, and sunflower oils are all acceptable alternatives. Note, however, that the antimicrobial properties of coconut may cause yeast infections in some women. Sesame oil, when used as a lubricant during intercourse, has been shown in some studies to impair sperm motility, and may impede fertility. Oils can also degrade the integrity of latex condoms, so they are not always compatible with safe sex and pregnancy prevention practices.

- ALOE VERA (Aloe barbadensis) is known as a topical remedy for minor burns and irritations, and is used as an ingredient in some over-the-counter (and chemically laden) lubricants. But 100% pure aloe vera, when combined with oils or applied directly to dry areas and tissues, is a superior choice.

- VITAMIN E oil and SEA BUCKTHORN oil also provide excellent moisturization. Both have been shown in some studies to have beneficial effects on vaginal health. They are also used as treatments for strengthening vaginal tissues in postmenopausal women (and those with other hormone-related issues). As with other oils, they can degrade the material used in condoms.

- Many commercial lubricants contain chemical 'warming' agents that can increase blood flow and sensitivity as well as temporarily providing moisture. The following natural essential oils are among those that women have come to rely on for finding balance and additional support in calming vaginal tissues and/or providing stimulation:

  - CALENDULA OIL – Used as an anti-inflammatory, with antiseptic properties.

  - CORIANDER – rich in antioxidants, complexion-friendly minerals and vitamin C.

  - CLARY SAGE – A world of uses, including as an antidepressant, antiseptic, aphrodisiac, astringent, bactericidal, carminative, and deodorant!

  - FRANKINCENSE – Stress-reliever, pain reducer, and a full-range skin care apothecary.

  - LAVENDER – Fragrant and calming, it's been used medicinally since ancient times.

  - NEROLI – Helps fight depression, an effective skin balm, and an antibacterial.

  - ORANGE - The fragrant extract can be used on sensitive, irritated skin.

  - PEPPERMINT – Invigorating and stimulating, great for the skin and hair.

- ROMAN CHAMOMILE – Promotes youthful-looking hair and skin, and combats insomnia.

- ROSE – Moisturizes skin, with antiseptic and astringent properties as well. Its anti-inflammatory properties help treat redness and inflammation.

- ROSEMARY – Contains a host of anti-inflammatory and antioxidant agents.

- SANDALWOOD – One of the most beneficial essential oils for skin and beauty use.

- THYME – Heals, protects, and naturally helps soothe and treat rashes.

- YLANG YLANG – Helps treat inflamed and dry skin.

Because of the potential for adverse reactions with the use of essential oils in the delicate vaginal area, care should be taken to select high-quality, therapeutic-grade oils, and to ensure they are properly diluted with carrier oils.

Oral medicinal herbs like Vitex (Chaste berry), Ashwagandha (Withania somnifera) and Shatavari (Asparagus racemosus) have also been shown to relieve vaginal dryness and menopausal symptoms. They often appear as treatment ingredients in Traditional Chinese Medicine (TCM) and Ayurveda.

Part 9: Oral Supplements for Skin and Female Health

Like our gut, the vagina is a sensitive ecosystem that contains a lot of good bacteria and yeasts. These bacteria create an acidic environment that helps our vaginas fight off infections and resist irritations. These beneficial live bacteria and yeasts (also called probiotics) help our entire immune system retain its strength, and our microbiome maintain its balance. Since about 80 percent of our immune system resides in our gut, imbalances in the microbiome can lead to many side effects including digestive issues, low energy, thyroid and autoimmune issues, and depression, to name just a few.

Inflammatory skin conditions like rosacea, psoriasis, eczema, and acne are often signs of an imbalance in the gut, and many of these conditions (including Candida and Bacterial Vaginosis) may be fixed when the gut microbiome is restored. Remember: When we treat the gut biome we treat the whole body, and the vaginal area benefits.

Regularly consuming yogurt, kefir (or non-dairy options), fermented foods, and supplementing these with a probiotic is often helpful in resolving gut issues, and may prevent new ones from occurring. Ideally, the probiotic will contain a minimum of 30 billion CFUs or 'colony forming units' in an acid-resistant capsule, so it is still viable after the trip through the acidic stomach. It should contain species of live cultures of Lactobacillus and Bifidobacterium, or be comprised of the less traditional (but increasingly popular) soil-based organisms (SBOs). The latter is argued to be superior, as the structure of SBOs is naturally resistant to the harsh environment of the upper digestive tract and stomach.

SUPPLEMENTS FOR SKIN IN GENERAL

Healthier skin is supported when the gut's microbiome is happy and the body is given the nourishment that it needs. Implementing a holistic approach to supplementation, and taking these supplements correctly and regularly along with a varied diet, is of paramount importance. When operating well, our bodies are designed to access all the nutrients they need from the food we eat. But even with probiotic use, most of us do not achieve a perfectly balanced diet and may want to consider supplements. Blood tests can be useful to reveal and understand where any deficiencies may exist. The list below includes vitamins and other additions that may aid overall skin health.

VITAMIN A – Supports healthy skin production and growth; keeps skin firm.

VITAMIN E – A moisturizing antioxidant that may help soften skin as well.

VITAMIN C – Essential in collagen production and maintenance, and a strong antioxidant that helps to neutralize free radicals in the skin.

VITAMIN D - Contributes to skin cell growth, repair, and metabolism.

B-COMPLEX – With Niacin (B3), this is a key ingredient for skin tone and health.

COENZYME Q10 – An antioxidant that helps skin cells stay vital and healthy.

CALCIUM – Mostly known for bone benefits, a lack of calcium can lead to thin and fragile skin.

ZINC – Helps heal the skin and regulate the function of oil glands.

COLLAGEN – An essential protein that provides elasticity to our skin.

MANGANESE – A natural mineral that serves as an antioxidant and neutralizes free radicals.

SELENIUM – As with vitamin E , Selenium helps to safeguard the protective coating around cells.

FISH OIL (krill, omega-3)/Flaxseed oil – These fatty oils help firm and plump the skin back to a more youthful appearance.
GLA oils (omega-6) Evening Primrose, Borage, Black Currant

OILS – These oils help hydrate, soothe, and nourish the skin.

ACAI – Helps revive skin, heal damaged skin cells, and restore moisture to skin and scalp.

BILBERRY – cleansing, tightening, and nourishing properties with antioxidants to help strengthen the skin.

MACA - Provides nutrients that nourish the endocrine system and regulate hormone levels. Traditionally used as an aphrodisiac.

ASHWAGANDHA - It is used to treat fatigue, and has a reputation as a strong aphrodisiac for both sexes,

ROSEHIP - With its concentration of antioxidants and Vitamins A and E, Rosehip Seed oil is known to support the skin's elasticity and promote healing.

GOJI BERRIES – Rich in antioxidants, vitamins, and minerals, its benefits include antioxidant and anti-aging protection, as well as improved skin tone.

MILK THISTLE - Found to have antioxidant and anti-aging effects on human skin cells

MSM – Soothes dry skin, guards against premature ageing and skin damage.

E3LIVE BLUE-GREEN ALGAE – A 'superfood' with a high concentration of protein, vitamins, trace minerals, and essential fatty acids.

GLUCOSAMINE – Improves skin hydration

CURCUMIN – Said to be beneficial in restoring the skin's natural glow.

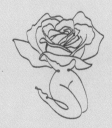

She knows that there is always a way. Her resilience and creativity, and her unwavering love of life, make her powerful.

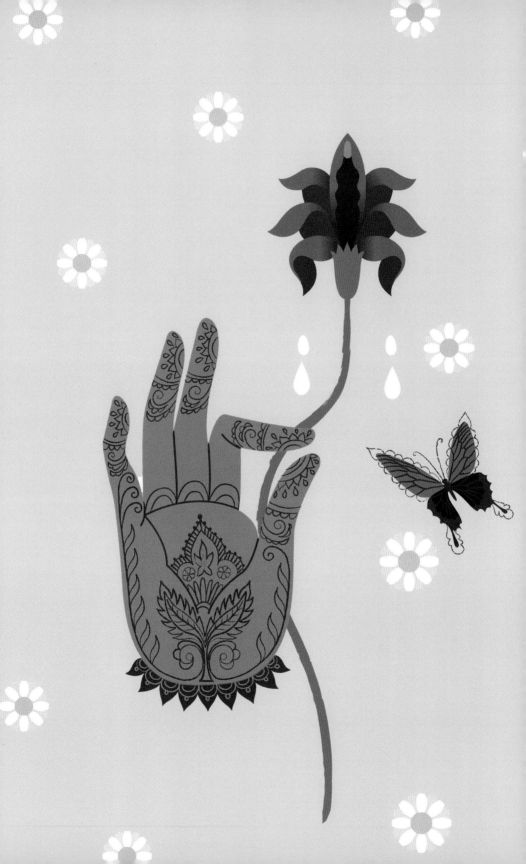

Part 10: A Lifetime of Joy and Self Love

To live our fullest lives, we can't hide from anything— especially our own bodies. When things move from shadow into light, and we accept and love ourselves in the places there once was shame, an ease takes over us, a joy and freedom. This isn't age dependent! The sooner we get in touch with self-love, transparency, and self-acceptance, the richer our overall quality of life will be. It's never too late.

Self-love can be simple. Treat yourself like you'd treat a lover! Wake up in the morning and touch your whole body. Give thanks for the mere experience of being alive, for another day on earth. Feed your body good food, take it for a good stretch and sweat. Take it out to play.

Honor your priorities as well. Learn to say "yes" with joy and "no" with a soft heart. Learn to walk away from people who are yelling or screaming at you. Ask for what you want, without expectation. Find your joy and what moves you and follow that compass, a little at a time if you need to—and then go at it full steam. That might mean a lot of hard, rewarding work to reach a place of mastery, or to create something impactful in the lives of others.

Joy isn't the same as pleasure. The point is: No one will give you permission to be your full self, no one can live your life for you. Even though we lean into community for mutual support and guidance, the spark of life is within us. We are the decider of our own destinies, within the limits of externalities and the social constructs we exist within.

We live wholly dependent on the sun and the air. We are nature itself. We are nature! Like a tree or a flower, we are born whole and perfect, and grow perfectly in tune with what's demanded of us, or what we demand of us. There is no way we cannot be enough. That goes for our minds, lives and bodies. Whether through circumstance, genetics, or choice, we grow as we should. The light and life force flows through us and animates us all the time: That's what we are at our core, and this awareness can fuel an even deeper appreciation for the miracle of sensory embodiment. We are both AND: we are the body that has sensory experience and will eventually die, and we are the inner nucleus that is unchanging and eternal.

In accepting this, and by integrating the two, we are neither in cultural or religious repressive denial about our sensual, physical selves, floating off into some aggrandized "spiritual life"—NOR are we some deadened meat body that thinks we ourselves are the source of our ideas and energy, isolated beings, anxiety laden and competitive and disconnected, objectifying our own bodies.

We invite you to do this: Live into the deepest possible experience of being alive in your body. Take some time to drop into your sensual nature. Get to know your feminine warrior: the one who knows what's right for you, and who knows what being "for life" really means. Feel your sex. Feel the intricate power of the biology of creating life. Feel the miracle of the fact that women are made to bring human life into the world, and love that truth whether you choose to have babies or not. Love the curves that come with that power, the curves that are designed to bear and nurture. Love your strong arms, back, and legs.

Perhaps your unique way of being human exists at the lower end of the continuum of valuing sensuality and sexuality. Some of us are made truly asexual, or with an aversion to touch. Some people may feel feminine without the body parts that match that conviction biologically. Even cisgender (a person whose sense of personal identity and gender corresponds with their birth sex) males can embrace the nurturing, receptive, creative parts in themselves, and come into a little softening, opening and expression—much like we, as women, can embrace our agency, strength, and power. Gender traits are an indeterminate blend of culture and biology, and they live in all of us, in varying degrees. Self love means accepting that. There is no one right way to be human.

In all of the decades and the passing years, we will change, the body will change. Love the changes too. Sensual pleasure doesn't end with aging.

If you have a vagina, look at it, get to know it, let it see the light of day, let it see the sun. Honor it as an integral part of you. Care for it, and respect it, like you would your heart or gut or brain or face. Bring this core of the feminine out of the shadows, literally and metaphorically.

To more freedom, power, clarity, grace, peace, compassion and love in each of us, and for all the world.

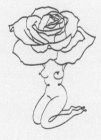

No soul is desolate as long as there is a human being
for whom it can feel trust and reverence.
- GEORGE ELIOT

ABOUT

Rosebud Woman™ is committed to awakening self love and reverence for the feminine in the world. We make luxury, plant based intimate skincare and body care that support women's common concerns. We are committed to natural ingredients, philanthropy and the highest standards in production and quality.

Find us at www.RoseWoman.com
@RosebudWoman on all social media channels.

Contributors to this volume:

CHRISTINE MARIE MASON

Founder of Rosebud Woman. Author. Yogi. Philosopher.
Find her at: www.rosewoman.com or www.XtineM.com

CAROLYN DAVIS

Researcher, writer, photographer, sexuality educator.
Find her at: www.CarolynEDavis.com

MARIA FINNA (OUVRA)

Australian artist specializing in empowerment art, with pussy portraits and nano love stories to life.
Find her at: www.instagram.com/ouvra

JEFF GREENWALD

Author, travel journalist, editor, performer, songwriter.
Find him at: www.jeffgreenwald.com

ROBERT SILBER

Global Educator in Human Connection, Sexuality and Tantra, founder of Lollia Place, host of the Hawaii Tantra Festival. Find him at: www.ConsciousSensuality.com

RESOURCES

To find out about known environmental toxins by zip code, check out:
http://scorecard.goodguide.com

To find out more about toxins in your skincare products, Skindeep, the Environmental Working Group's cosmetics database.
https://www.ewg.org/skindeep/

Anatomy Sources
https://www.healthline.com/health/mons-pubis#What's-the-anatomy-and-function-of-the-mons-pubis?
http://www.bumc.bu.edu/sexualmedicine/physicianinformation/female-genital-anatomy/

https://www.sciencedirect.com/topics/medicine-and-dentistry/clitoris

https://www.ncbi.nlm.nih.gov/pubmed/16145367

https://www.sciencedirect.com/topics/veterinary-science-and-veterinary-medicine/labia-minora

https://www.ourbodiesourselves.org/book-excerpts/health-article/self-exam-vulva-vagina/

http://www.bumc.bu.edu/sexualmedicine/physicianinformation/female-genital-anatomy/

https://www.niddk.nih.gov/health-information/urologic-diseases/urinary-tract-how-it-works